Corine J. Williamson

The Erotic Mind

How Your Thoughts Affect Your Sexual Experiences

Copyright © 2023 by Corine J. Williamson

About the book

The Erotic Mind refers to the role that our thoughts and beliefs play in shaping our sexual experiences. Our minds have the power to influence how we perceive our bodies, our partners, and our sexual experiences, and can impact our levels of arousal, satisfaction, and pleasure. In this chapter, we will explore the importance of understanding and cultivating a positive erotic mind, and the impact it can have on our overall sexual well-being.

Our beliefs and expectations play a significant role in how we experience sexuality. Positive beliefs and expectations can lead to increased pleasure, while negative beliefs and expectations can lead to anxiety, shame, and even sexual dysfunction. In this chapter, we will explore the ways in which beliefs and expectations can impact our sexual experiences, and how we can cultivate positive beliefs and expectations to enhance our sexual well-being.

Body image and sexual self-esteem are crucial components of our erotic mind. Negative body image can lead to decreased sexual desire, while positive body image can enhance sexual pleasure and satisfaction. In this chapter, we will explore the impact of body image on sexual self-esteem and discuss strategies for cultivating a positive body image and enhancing sexual self-esteem.

Communication and connection are essential for healthy and satisfying sexual experiences. Our ability to communicate our desires and boundaries, and to connect with our partners on an emotional level, can significantly impact our sexual experiences. In this chapter, we will explore the role of communication and connection in sexuality, and discuss strategies for enhancing both.

Mindfulness and presence are key components of the erotic mind. Being present and fully engaged in our sexual experiences can enhance pleasure and satisfaction, while distracted or disengaged thinking can detract from it. In this chapter, we will explore the benefits of mindfulness and presence in sexuality, and discuss strategies for cultivating these qualities in our erotic mind.

Fantasies and imagination are powerful tools for enhancing sexual pleasure and satisfaction. Our minds have the ability to create vivid and exciting scenarios that can increase arousal and satisfaction. In this chapter, we will explore the role of fantasies and imagination in sexuality, and discuss strategies for using them to enhance our sexual experiences.

Sexual trauma can have a profound impact on our erotic mind. Trauma can lead to negative beliefs and expectations, decreased sexual desire, and even sexual dysfunction. In this chapter, we will explore the impact of sexual trauma on sexuality, and discuss strategies for healing and reclaiming our sexual well-being.

Cultivating a positive erotic mind requires ongoing attention and effort. In this chapter, we will explore strategies for cultivating a positive erotic mind, including self-reflection, self-compassion, and self-care. We will also discuss the benefits of seeking professional support when needed.

Table of contents

Introduction to the Erotic Mind

The erotic mind refers to the complex psychological and emotional processes that underlie human sexuality and sexual desire. It encompasses the thoughts, feelings, and fantasies that arise in response to sexual stimuli, as well as the ways in which individuals navigate their own sexual identities, preferences, and boundaries.

The erotic mind is shaped by a variety of factors, including biology, culture, personal experience, and individual personality traits. For example, research has shown that certain brain regions, such as the amygdala and the hypothalamus, are closely involved in the processing of sexual stimuli and the regulation of sexual behavior.

Culture also plays a significant role in shaping the erotic mind. Societal norms and values around sex and sexuality can influence what individuals find arousing, how they express their desires, and what types of sexual experiences they feel comfortable exploring.

Personal experience and individual personality traits also contribute to the formation of the erotic mind. Past sexual experiences, as well as feelings of shame or guilt around sex, can impact an individual's sexual desire and behavior. Additionally, personality traits such as openness, extraversion, and neuroticism have been linked to differences in sexual attitudes and behaviors.

Overall, understanding the erotic mind is crucial for individuals seeking to explore and understand their own sexual desires and preferences, as well as for researchers and clinicians seeking to better understand and treat sexual dysfunction and other sexual health concerns.

The Power of Beliefs and Expectations

Beliefs and expectations are powerful forces that shape our thoughts, feelings, and behaviors. They are the lenses through which we view the world and interpret our experiences. Our beliefs and expectations can be both positive and negative, and they can have a profound impact on our lives.

Positive beliefs and expectations can empower us and help us achieve our goals. They can give us the confidence to take on challenges, and the motivation to persist in the face of obstacles. For example, if you believe that you are capable of achieving success in your career, you are more likely to work hard, persevere through setbacks, and eventually reach your goals.

Negative beliefs and expectations, on the other hand, can limit us and hold us back. They can create a sense of self-doubt, anxiety, and fear that prevents us from taking risks and pursuing our dreams. For example, if you believe that you are not good enough to achieve your goals, you may be less likely to try, and you may give up more easily when faced with difficulties.

It's important to recognize that our beliefs and expectations are not fixed, and can be changed with effort and practice. By becoming aware of our negative beliefs and expectations, we can challenge them and replace them with more positive and empowering ones. This can involve questioning the evidence that supports our negative beliefs, seeking out alternative perspectives, and practicing new ways of thinking and behaving.

Beliefs and expectations can have a significant impact on a person's sexuality. These beliefs and expectations can come from a variety of sources, including cultural, social, religious, and personal experiences.

One of the ways that beliefs and expectations can influence sexuality is by shaping a person's understanding of what is considered "normal" or "acceptable" sexual behavior. For example, a person who grew up in a conservative religious community may have been taught that certain sexual behaviors, such as premarital sex or homosexuality, are sinful or immoral. This belief can lead to feelings of guilt or shame surrounding sexuality, which can in turn impact a person's sexual experiences and relationships.

Beliefs and expectations can also affect a person's sexual desire and arousal. For instance, if a person believes that they are not attractive or desirable, they may struggle with feeling sexually confident or initiating sexual activity. On the other hand, if a person has positive beliefs and expectations about their own sexual abilities or attractiveness, they may feel more comfortable exploring their sexuality and expressing their desires.

Moreover, cultural beliefs and expectations can also impact how people view gender roles and sexual orientation. For example, a society that values traditional gender roles may view heterosexual relationships as the norm, while same-sex relationships may be stigmatized or seen as abnormal. These cultural beliefs and expectations can influence a person's own beliefs and attitudes about their sexual identity, which can affect their behavior and relationships.

Overall, beliefs and expectations play a crucial role in shaping a person's sexuality. By recognizing and understanding how these beliefs and expectations impact us, we can work towards developing a healthier and more fulfilling sexual identity.

Body Image and Sexual Self-Esteem

Body image refers to the mental representation an individual has of their physical appearance. It includes their perceptions, thoughts, and feelings about their body and how they believe others perceive them. Body image can be influenced by a variety of factors, including cultural standards of beauty, media images, social interactions, and personal experiences.

Sexual self-esteem, on the other hand, refers to the level of confidence and satisfaction an individual has with their sexual self-concept, including their sexual feelings, behaviors, and desires. Sexual self-esteem can be influenced by a range of factors, including body image, sexual experiences, cultural norms and values, and social support.

Research has shown that there is a strong correlation between body image and sexual self-esteem. Individuals who have a positive body image tend to have higher levels of sexual self-esteem, while those with negative body image tend to have lower levels of sexual self-esteem. This is because body image can influence how individuals feel about themselves and their ability to engage in sexual activities.

For example, individuals with negative body image may feel self-conscious or ashamed during sexual activities, which can lead to lower levels of sexual satisfaction and lower sexual self-esteem. On the other hand, individuals with positive body image may feel more comfortable and confident during sexual activities, leading to higher levels of sexual satisfaction and higher sexual self-esteem.

It is important to note that body image and sexual self-esteem can be influenced by a variety of factors, and addressing these issues often requires a multifaceted approach. This may include therapy, counseling, social support, and other interventions designed to improve body image and sexual self-esteem. By working to improve both body image and sexual self-esteem, individuals can experience greater sexual satisfaction and a more positive overall sense of self.

Communication and Connection

Communication and connection are essential components of a healthy sexual relationship. Effective communication involves the ability to express one's thoughts and feelings about sexual desires, preferences, and boundaries, as well as the ability to listen and respond to one's partner's needs and desires.

Communication can involve verbal and nonverbal cues, such as body language and tone of voice. It can also include sharing fantasies, exploring new ideas, and discussing sexual experiences. By openly communicating about sexual desires and boundaries, partners can build trust, respect, and intimacy with one another.

Connection in sexuality refers to the emotional and physical bond between partners. It involves creating a safe and comfortable environment where both partners can freely express themselves and explore their desires. Connection can be achieved through physical touch, eye contact, and intimacy, such as hugging, kissing, and cuddling.

Connection can also be built through shared experiences and activities, such as exploring new sexual positions, trying new toys, and experimenting with different forms of foreplay. Through shared experiences, partners can develop a deeper understanding of each other's desires and build a stronger bond.

In summary, communication and connection are integral to a healthy sexual relationship. By openly communicating and building emotional and physical connections with one another, partners can create a fulfilling and satisfying sexual experience.

Mindfulness and Presence

Mindfulness and presence are powerful tools that can enhance our experiences in all areas of life, including sexuality. When we practice mindfulness and presence during sexual experiences, we can fully engage our senses and connect with our bodies and partners in a more profound way.

Mindfulness is the practice of being fully present in the moment, without judgment or distraction. This can be applied to sexuality by bringing attention to our bodies, our sensations, and our emotions. By being mindful during sexual experiences, we can notice and appreciate the subtle sensations and nuances of pleasure, as well as any discomfort or tension that may arise.

Presence, on the other hand, is the state of being fully engaged and connected to our surroundings and the people around us. When we practice presence during sexual experiences, we can deepen our connections with our partners and fully immerse ourselves in the pleasure and intimacy of the moment.

In terms of sexuality, mindfulness and presence can help us to better understand our own bodies and desires, as well as those of our partners. By being fully present and attentive, we can learn to communicate more effectively with our partners, expressing our needs and desires in a way that is both respectful and assertive.

In addition, mindfulness and presence can help us to overcome any anxiety or shame we may feel about our sexuality. By being fully present in the moment and accepting our bodies and desires without judgment, we can cultivate a greater sense of self-acceptance and self-love.

Overall, mindfulness and presence are powerful tools that can help us to cultivate more fulfilling and satisfying sexual experiences. By being fully present and attentive, we can deepen our connections with our bodies and partners, and unlock new levels of pleasure and intimacy.

Fantasies and Imagination

Fantasies and imagination are both powerful tools of the human mind that allow us to create worlds and experiences that may not exist in reality. Imagination is the ability to form mental images or concepts of things that are not physically present or have not been experienced before. It involves the use of our senses to create mental representations of ideas, thoughts, and sensations.

On the other hand, fantasies are elaborate and unrealistic scenarios or stories that are created in our minds. They often involve characters, events, and situations that may not be possible in reality, and they can be based on desires, fears, or any other aspects of our inner lives. Fantasies can be harmless and fun, like daydreaming about winning the lottery, or they can be more complex and even disturbing, like imagining extreme scenarios of violence or revenge.

Both imagination and fantasy are crucial to our creativity, problem-solving abilities, and emotional well-being. They can help us explore new ideas and perspectives, cope with difficult situations, and express our deepest desires and fears. In childhood, imagination and fantasy play a significant role in cognitive and social development, as children use their creativity to make sense of the world around them and develop social skills through pretend play.

However, it's important to note that while imagination and fantasy can be positive and productive, they can also be detrimental if taken too far. Obsessive or delusional fantasies can lead to mental health issues, and relying too heavily on imagination can cause us to disconnect from reality and neglect important aspects of our lives. It's crucial to maintain a healthy balance between reality and fantasy, and to use our imaginations in a constructive and responsible way.

Sexual Trauma and Healing

Sexual trauma refers to any unwanted or non-consensual sexual experience that can cause significant distress, shame, and other negative emotional reactions. Sexual trauma can occur at any point in a person's life, and can take many different forms, including sexual assault, rape, sexual harassment, and molestation.

Healing from sexual trauma is a complex and deeply personal process that can take time, patience, and support. There are many different approaches to healing from sexual trauma, and what works best for one person may not work for another.

One common approach to healing from sexual trauma is therapy, which can provide a safe space for survivors to process their experiences, develop coping skills, and work through the emotions and behaviors that may be associated with their trauma. Different types of therapy may be more effective for different people, and may include cognitive-behavioral therapy, trauma-focused therapy, and somatic therapy.

Another important aspect of healing from sexual trauma is building a supportive network of friends, family, and professionals who can offer validation, empathy, and practical assistance. Support groups and advocacy organizations can also provide valuable resources and opportunities for connection with other survivors.

Physical self-care can also be an important part of the healing process, as survivors may experience physical symptoms such as pain, tension, or dissociation as a result of their trauma. Practicing mindfulness, yoga, and other relaxation techniques can help survivors to reconnect with their bodies and develop a sense of safety and comfort.

Ultimately, healing from sexual trauma is a unique and ongoing journey that requires compassion, patience, and a commitment to self-care. While the effects of sexual trauma can be long-lasting, with the right support and resources, survivors can learn to reclaim their power and live fulfilling lives.

Cultivating a Positive Erotic Mind

Cultivating a positive erotic mind refers to developing a healthy and empowering relationship with one's sexuality and sexual thoughts. This involves creating an environment of positivity and openness towards one's own sexual desires and fantasies, and learning to embrace and express them in a healthy and consensual manner.

The process of cultivating a positive erotic mind involves developing a sense of self-awareness, understanding one's sexual preferences and boundaries, and working towards self-acceptance and self-love. It also involves learning to communicate effectively about one's sexual desires and needs with partners and practicing enthusiastic consent.

Practicing self-care and self-love is an important aspect of cultivating a positive erotic mind. This includes engaging in activities that promote self-confidence, self-esteem, and positive body image, such as exercise, meditation, and therapy. It also involves avoiding negative self-talk and limiting beliefs that may hinder one's sexual expression and pleasure.

Additionally, cultivating a positive erotic mind involves developing healthy and respectful relationships with sexual partners. This includes practicing open and honest communication, establishing boundaries and expectations, and prioritizing consent and respect.

Overall, cultivating a positive erotic mind is a lifelong journey of self-discovery and self-acceptance. It involves embracing one's sexual desires and fantasies without shame or judgment, and learning to express them in a healthy and empowering way that respects oneself and others.

About the Author

The Erotic Mind: How Your Thoughts Affect Your Sexual Experiences" is a book written by Corine J. Williamsona, clinical psychologist and sex therapist. The book explores the connection between the mind and the body in regards to sexual experiences. Williamsona argues that our thoughts and beliefs about sex and sexuality have a profound impact on our sexual experiences.

One of the key conclusions of the book is that our sexual experiences are shaped by our beliefs and attitudes about sex. For example, if we have negative beliefs or attitudes about sex, such as shame or guilt, it can lead to sexual dysfunction, dissatisfaction, or avoidance. On the other hand, positive beliefs and attitudes can enhance sexual experiences and lead to greater intimacy and connection with our partners.

Williamsona also emphasizes the importance of understanding and exploring our sexual fantasies and desires. He argues that our fantasies can reveal important information about our sexual selves and can be a healthy way to explore our desires. However, he cautions that we should not confuse fantasy with reality and that it is important to communicate our fantasies and desires with our partners in a consensual and respectful manner.

Overall, "The Erotic Mind" provides a valuable insight into the complex and multifaceted nature of human sexuality. It highlights the importance of understanding and exploring our own beliefs and attitudes about sex and sexuality, and how they can impact our sexual experiences. By doing so, we can cultivate a healthier and more fulfilling sexual life.

9 798388 519351